MW01195886

THE BOOK OF BALD
GOING BALD LIKE A MAN

ISBN 9781726747202
www.bookofbald.com.

SETTING THE RECORD STRAIGHT

I'm not a doctor and I'm not a scientist. I'm no expert on minoxidil or finasteride. I'm just a bald guy with some opinions.

As a man, these opinions aren't always rooted in fact. I didn't write this book asking for directions, I navigated the sun and took my shit off-road.

If you're looking for interviews with PhDs and other bookworms, this isn't your drink.

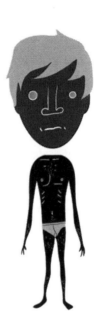

SYMP-TOM

noun

"a sign of the existence of something, especially of

an undesirable situation"

The Seed

"You're losing your hair."

I squint and smirk, a little confused and a little surprised. "What?" I snort. "No I'm not."

Nick reaches over the neck of his acoustic and grabs his beer off my desk. "Yeah, dude, you're gonna be bald," he says. "Your bangs are getting all stringy."

I shake my head, catching my reflection in the laptop, then brush my bangs to the side. They're fine.

"This is stupid," says Nick. "It's Friday. Why the hell is everyone studying?" He grabs the laptop and balances it on his knee, pecking the keys with his free hand, as though he's said nothing.

My bangs are long and flipped to the side to stay out of my eyes. Nowadays people call it the *Beiber*, but I've been doing it for years. I call it the *Weber*.

"I know what you're trying to do, man. I've got more hair than you do."

"Dude, who cares?" Nick mumbles, entranced by Facebook. "Wear a hat or something."

Nick has the demeanor of a caffeine tweeker, all jerky and spazzy with the angular face of a lizard. He has thick black hair that always seems wet, adding to his reptilian appearance. He's A.D.D. as fuck and can't go a second without some sort of stimulus, like trying to get a rise out of me with his festering comments.

"You're an ass," I laugh, grabbing the Pabst at my foot.

He laughs through his nose and says nothing.

I run my fingers through my hair again. It's straight and auburn with blondish-red highlights spiraling from the crown. My mom loves the colour and says anyone would kill for it. But she's my mom. Others say I'm a ginger.

"Wanna go downtown?" Nick slurs. "I got a message from Michelle. She and Lauren are going to Chinatown to get fake IDs."

"Sure," I say. "Gimme a second."

I get up and shuffle past Nick to the washroom, take a leak and step to the sink. I splash my face with water, then wet my hair and dry it with a towel. Lately, I've been going for that careless, messy look.

Stringy, I think to myself. *I guess it could be a bit thicker.*

I brush my hair to the left and can't help feeling a subtle sinking in my chest. *Has there always been that much skin peeking through? When did I start parting it like this? Why did I start parting it like this?*

I look at the insecure freshman in the mirror.

"You're too easy," I laugh. "This is what Nick does."

The confidence leaves my body as soon as the words leave my lips. It's that feeling you get when you're on a plane and hit turbulence. "Tell my wife I love her!" you joke, but when the plane keeps rocking there's that uneasy voice whispering, "*Well, plane crashes do happen . . .*"

"Well, some people *do* go bald," I said, that night and every night for the next three years. Every morning, after every shower, after every shit . . . In the reflection of every window, my cell screen, my laptop. Three years of turbulence. Three years counting hairs on my pillow every morning. Three years getting haircuts and saying, "Don't take any off the top." Three years to go from Justin Beiber to George Costanza. Three years to . . .

I'm getting ahead of myself. This is supposed to be a book, not a suicide note . . . though increasingly, it feels like a fine line.

Fine, like the hairs you'll dust off the sink after a Buzzcut.

Fine, what your girlfriend says when you bail on brunch.

Fine . . . how you're going to feel when it's all over.

******

I never thought I'd go bald. Yeah, John Weber, my dad, is bald, but I grew up understanding that the bald gene comes from your mom's side. In my case, Grandpa Lloyd had been rocking the Elvis since the great depression so I figured I had nothing to worry about. Throw in the fact that Johnny Bald was the only cue ball in the entire family tree, I was more than comfortable making jokes at his expense.

There was the classic head buff to see my reflection and the whole crystal ball routine. That's the real joke: a crystal ball would have told me to stop being an ass. Karma was coming.

Maybe I made one too many jokes about his glaring dome shooting hoops in the driveway. Still, despite the jabs, I never thought he looked weird. Bald suited my dad. You know those guys like Vin Diesel who look like they were never meant to have hair? That's my dad. I've tried imagining him with the long, blonde locks he sported in the 70's and it's just weird. He's got a well-shaped skull with no bumps or crevices, not one of those brainy-looking alien heads. His was meant to be flaunted. Beyond his appearance, he's always had fun with his hair loss, claiming, "If I had hair I'd be too good looking, it just wouldn't be fair."

Genetics aside, knowing my fate wouldn't change anything, because *predicting* bald and *going* bald are entirely different. If you're growing up in a fat family, you can assume you'll be overweight but it doesn't mean you'll to be at peace with man-boobs, chaffing thighs, or the *what-the-fuck* number on your scale.

Balding or not, one thing that will help is knowing you'll still have the relationships in life that are most important. You'll still have your girlfriend who loves you, *right?* . . . even when you start looking like Gollum. You'll still have your friends . . . unless you become a total buzzkill, a dickless shell of a man who can't keep up chasing girls. Your hairline might wedge itself between you and your family, your co-workers, and your sense of self . . . Okay, okay, shit might get dark but at least you'll have the bald brotherhood to build you back up. Truth is, we've lost a lot of good men. We don't want to lose you too.

And that's the point of this book. *I've* made the journey and come back for you. Let me be your hairless Sherpa. It's a slippery slope but I'll show you the way.

Sometimes life cracks you on the chin and you buckle. Sometimes you might drop, but this is about getting back up! It's not gonna be easy, but that's what being a real man is about. And you're a real man, I *know* it. You *have* to be a real man, 'cause balding is linked to god-like levels of testosterone! Stone Cold Steve Austin is bald for fuck sakes!

If anyone can beat hair loss it's you.

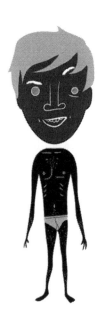

DE-NI-AL

noun

"the action of declaring something to be untrue"

I raise my eyebrows and scrunch my forehead like I'm surprised or scared. I count three horizontal wrinkles, run a sharpie from the top wrinkle to my hairline, then measure with my index and middle fingers. Holding my bangs back, I snap a photo with my webcam.

One and three quarters of an inch; maybe one and a half.

I tongue the inside of my cheek while inspecting the

photo. I look back in the mirror at my scribbled forehead.

Delete

I raise my eyebrows and scrunch my forehead even more, struggling to create a fourth wrinkle. I hold the expression just long enough, mark it and snap.

One and a quarter, give or take.

I type "June, 2010", click *Save As*, then open "May, 2010" to compare the images. I sigh with relief like an addict after a hit.

I'm not balding . . . just going crazy.

What am I doing, you ask? Only the most advanced self-diagnostic balding procedure this side of the internet. It might seem a little archaic and unreliable, using markers and finger widths to track the distance between my hairline and forehead wrinkles. Sure, my forehead could be getting more wrinkly over time, and the tilt of my head is slightly different in each photo. Maybe my fingers don't perfectly measure an inch, but *MensHairForum.com* gave this method their seal of approval so it's good enough for me. Unverified studies show that if your hairline remains two finger widths higher than your top forehead wrinkle, you're not dying . . . er, I mean, going bald. It's *SCIENCE*, goddammit! Who am I to doubt the anonymous posters of online forums?

Give it a try! Find a mirror, raise your eyebrows as high as you can, say a prayer and measure. Is it more than two finger widths? Is it less?

What's that you say? The only people posting on *MensHairForum.com* are schmucks obsessing over hair loss? That if you're drawing lines on your face every month you're a total psycho? A *balding* psycho?

Truthfully, you'll only find these half-baked tactics if you're researching male pattern baldness. That's the real test: if you're looking for ways to see if you're losing your hair, *you're probably losing your fucking hair!*

HAIRLINE MEASURING

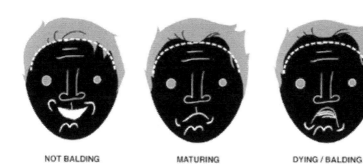

NOT BALDING   MATURING   DYING / BALDING

The forehead wrinkle test is specifically used to determine whether your hairline is receding or maturing. Now, only the luckiest guys keep their teenage hairline long term, while everyone else develops a mature hairline, one that slowly recedes then eventually stops. Yours might recede just enough to make you sweat, but probably not enough to make you actually work on yourself.

When Nick first chirped me, I was twenty-two years

old, midway through my second year of a Visual Arts degree at University of Toronto.

I was tall and skinny with pale skin, blue eyes and the same Beiber flow I described earlier. Despite the mental image this probably creates, I considered myself a soft 7, the essence of average.

Now, I've never had a problem being average. At a party I could talk to pretty girls without looking lost, hang with the quirky losers without it seeming like charity, and if the music wasn't too loud, probably talk a girl into making out with me. I've never tormented myself drooling over unattainable women and don't get too bent out of shape when certain opportunities in life seem out of reach. I'm not the athlete and I'm not the pretty boy. I'm average—a content 7—and I'm okay with that.

But the threat of dropping to a 6 was always in the back of my mind. With my frame and a less-than-baller future in the arts, going bald would likely knock me down to a 4—or even a 3—so I was all in on this "mature hairline" shit.

Here's why.

The maturing hairline is the "big boned" of balding and will be your go-to move when shit gets hot. For example, when Nick says your bangs are stringy you'll fire back with a blitz on mature hairlines: "Yeah? Well how many adults do you see brushing the hair out of their eyes? It's called a mature hairline, bro. Read a book."

You can even take it a step further, using your hair's maturity to question that of your peers. Like, "Good, I was getting tired of looking like a fifteen-year-old. It's a maturing hairline. How's puberty treating you?"

This was my go-to through my first year of balding,

something like "Nah, I've just got a mature hairline. My Grandpa has one too, an' he's *still rockin'* a full head of hair."

See how I worked in the genetics too? I kept it light, but factual. This preserved my 7 status and kept any doubts at bay. While it wasn't fool-proof, when things got dicey I could always fall back on my flawless crown.

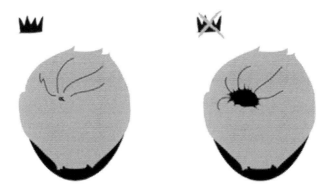

Besides the receding hairline, the most obvious sign of balding is a blown-to-shit crown, like and island of skin in a sea of hair. However, a thinning crown has another name that instills hope and optimism as you stare down the barrel of the gun:

The Bald Spot.

Now, technically it *is* a bald spot but by definition then, don't all bald men just have really large bald spots? These days, couldn't I claim my entire head is just one big bald spot?

The lie is in the implied harmlessness of the term, as though a bald spot is like a skin irritation you just brush off because skin gets weird sometimes. A true bald spot is what you get when your friends attack you with a beard trimmer, not what's hiding under your uncle's ball cap. They're like double agents, waiting for you to drop your guard. Then, before you know it you're bagged and tied up under a spotlight.

You probably first noticed your bald spot in the shower or after the back of your head got tagged in a photo. You ignored it because you didn't feel like you were balding, as though balding should come with a sore throat or some feeling of malaise. Maybe you thought of your head as a garden, with a small barren section always in the shade, near the back. Maybe that part of your head just doesn't grow hair, you'll think. That's totally different from balding, *right*? It's not like you see the back of your head all the time. Maybe it's always been like that?

It's funny. Regardless how enormous your crop circle is, you'll find comfort in the idea it's always been there; that it's not getting worse.

In fact, if you start counting hairs on your pillow each morning like I did, you'll lie about that, too. One morning you'll count five hairs, the next you'll count eight. Instead of curling up and dying you'll convince yourself you must have missed some the day before; that it's always been eight. It sounds crazy—because eight is more than five, right?—but the fact that it's always been eight will make you feel better, like losing the same number each night makes it normal. You'll probably go so far as to run a Google search: *How many hairs do you lose at night?* and find a million different answers, but as soon as one of them is eight, you'll be golden.

Crazy, I know. No, literally, it *is* crazy; like the behavior of a crazy person. *You'll be golden?* More likely, you'll be cross-eyed, tweezing hairs from your pillow, tallying them in blood on your headboard! You'll have smeared sharpie lines scribbled across your forehead as you spin around trying to see the back of your own head! All this while screaming about your mature hairline and your grandpa's genes!

The denial stage is like walking a tightrope, with rebuttals like your mature hairline and bald spot serving as balancing tools to keep you from falling. And that steadfast believe your hair's always looked a certain way? Nothing more than illusion, seeing the tightrope as a bridge, keeping you from looking down.

Now, sadly, when denial becomes your go-to move, it's clear you're on a sinking ship. What happens when you measure three fingers instead of two, or you count twenty hairs the day after you counted eight? You can only lie to yourself so long. What happens when you look down and your illusory bridge suddenly disappears?

For me, the illusion died one day in second-year painting class. The theme of the project was *"Self As . . . "*, where students were tasked with creating portraits of themselves as certain characters (i.e. *"Self as Matador", "Self as Vampire"*). I was going for some Godfather mafioso vibe, so I threw on a suit jacket, made a plate of spaghetti and slicked back my hair . . .

Good Lord!

By this time, I'd fallen off with the hairline tracking and hadn't brushed back my stringy bangs for months. Needless to say, my hairline had moved up and back like the visor of a motorcycle helmet.

Nothing from *MensHairForum* could rationalize the eggshell hiding under my crabgrass of a haircut. Instantly, I felt it in my stomach, the same feeling I had when I first noticed my stringy bangs. The feeling you get when your girlfriend texts, "We need to talk . . . " The feeling of your own mortality. The feeling you're . . . *caught.* I'd been living in denial for well over a year and already it felt like a lifetime ago.

17

Because it was.

I felt my former life slipping through my fingers like fine hairs through a comb. I wasn't the same guy anymore, casually flipping hair from his eyes while shredding guitar. Now, I was the guy brushing five different ways for maximum coverage; vulnerable to wind, scared of the rain.

In a flash it was clear. I was, in fact, losing my hair. But the deception continued. *As long as I keep my bangs long,* I thought, *I can still fly under the radar.*

I was like the guy who gets bit in the zombie movie but keeps it to himself. Sweaty and agitated, I could feel myself changing . . .

If I stay level-headed, I thought, *keep moving forward . . . maybe, just maybe, I can get in front of this thing . . .*

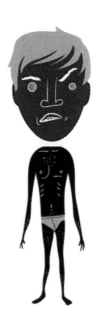

RE-SIST-ANCE

noun

"the refusal to accept or comply with something; the attempt to prevent something by action or argument"

"Excuse me . . ."

The woman stops and smiles, grocery-store friendly. "Hi, what can I do for you?"

"I'm looking for extra virgin olive oil . . . can't seem to find it here . . ."

"Hmm," she says, stepping forward, skimming the various bottles lining the shelf.

"We don't seeeeeem . . . to haaaaave annyyyyyyy," she mumbles, running her finger across the shelf like she was checking in brail.

"But, we do have this," she says before handing me a tall skinny bottle of virgin olive oil. "It's basically the same."

I skim the label, thinking back to everything I read earlier.

"Maybe you have some extra virgin oil in the back?"

She squints, shaking her head. "Sorry hun, this is all the olive oil we have, but it'll work just fine. Tastes just the same."

I tell her thanks but no thanks and return the bottle to the shelf. The website specifically said "extra virgin".

"Actually," I blurt out, stopping the woman again, "maybe you can help me. My uhh, girlfriend puts this oil in her hair for a little extra volume. She massages it into her scalp before she showers or something? Supposedly does something for thin hair, I don't really know . . . she asked if I would grab some while I was out."

The woman nods, assuring me they only have what's on the shelf, totally oblivious to my motivation.

"Right. But in regards to hair, do you think there's much difference between the extra virgin and the regular virgin in terms of reducing the production of DHT? Like, do you think it's the extra virgins that do the trick?"

Judging by her reaction—and her hair—the woman had never thought of olive oil this way, let alone what those extra virgins were up to. Maybe it was stupid to go to Food Basics with hair questions? Maybe I should have hit a salon instead? Maybe I should have asked the woman with some friggin' volume instead of Miss Frizzle? Rookie mistake.

Regardless, I buy the virgin olive oil, telling the cashier my girlfriend will just have to hope for the best.

I return home and dart for my room like a kid buying condoms. I open my laptop to *Hairlosshelp.com* and go over the instructions one more time.

1) Wash and rinse hair with a mild shampoo to clean your scalp.

2) Apply half an ounce of extra virgin olive oil directly to your hair.

3) Let the oil soak for approx. 5 minutes.

4) Repeat step 1.

5) Disregard the fact that your insecurities have led you to bathing in cooking oil. Close your eyes and dream about your future hair.

This is all worth it.

I continued with the olive oil for several weeks with zero results. *Maybe the extra virgins do do the trick?* I shouldn't say there were no results, my skin became silky smooth and I was eating less fried foods.

Better skin and a better diet is nice, but it's not enough to handle the the humiliation.

The biggest struggle with the olive oil was mental. As a guy, I'm not supposed to care about superficial shit like hair. Obviously guys *do* care, but we're not allowed to show it because it goes against everything we understand as manly. Of course we're supposed to look good, but for some reason when we go the extra mile to make it happen it's written off as being metrosexual or feminine.

Think about it, when was the last time you trimmed your eyebrows? Now, when was the last time you trimmed your eyebrows and told someone about it?

You can blame women all you want, but truthfully, we do it to ourselves. We've all got that friend who shaves his chest or spends too long getting ready and we break his balls! We hate that guy! He's a pussy, a *Nancy*! We devolve into back-woods fucks, bashing each other for going the extra mile with our appearance. I remember ripping my roommate for wearing white pants! Meanwhile, I'm hiding olive oil in a plastic bag under the sink like it's a murder weapon! That's fucked up!

It's this principle that makes commercials for hair transplants and hair growth formulas so pathetic. You know the ones, some fat fuck named Steve doesn't have his shit together. He's got the weirdest balding pattern you've ever seen and for some reason, can't take a photo with proper lighting.

But then, he sells out and gets plugs.

Suddenly, Steve's grinning like Hasselhoff, playing touch football on the beach with his hot wife. The sun slowly sets, silhouetting his mullet flapping in the wind like Superman's cape. Cue the logo!

We hate Steve, not because he cares about his appearance but because he shows he cares. He's stepping out of the male mold, wilting to the same insecurities we can't bear to address ourselves. Does that make us cowards? Sure, but it also makes us men. And what's more important, your hair or your manhood?

Unfortunately, when you're facing hair loss it's more than a rhetorical question.

Balding makes you insecure and that makes you desperate. So, before you go answering the question, let's take a look at Steve's wonderful life when the cameras aren't rolling.

After he has sex with his bangin' wife, Steve wants nothing more than to roll over and sleep. But instead, he has to get out of bed and face the cold tile of his bathroom floor to reapply his minoxidil. This means Mrs. Steve misses out on the post-coital cuddling she so desperately needs. And what happens when she feels neglected night after night, shafted and alone?

Hope you like the couch!

Meanwhile, Steve has to wait twenty long minutes for his formula to set, so he sits on the toilet, flipping through his wife's magazines. It's the longest fifteen minutes of the day. His back aches from football, and he has to be up early to get that overtime pay. *Mrs. Steve's designer hand bags don't pay for themselves.*

Twenty minutes later, he's tip-toeing into the bedroom like a cat burglar so to not wake Mrs. Steve. Obviously that doesn't work, as she tosses and turns aggressively to let him know she's annoyed. On top of that, she's having PTSD flashbacks to when her first husband used to sneak home late after shacking up with his secretary. What happens when this irrational aggression and distain snowballs?

Someone's making his own breakfast.

In this scenario we assume Steve has a sex life at all, despite the very real chance he's been chemically neutered. There have been reports of men losing their ability to perform after using medications containing finasteride. A lot of good that experiment on your head is gonna do if you can't lay pipe, bucko.

Even if Steve's lucky enough to avoid any side effects, there's still the mental fallout from staving off the aging process.

For example, when Steve crawls onto his wife, all she sees is an old man disguised as his younger self, reminding her of her own aging. *How could anyone find me attractive,* she thinks, *with this weight, these wrinkles? Did Steve get the treatment for me or that new intern at his office? She's only twenty-two!*

All this while Steve's trying to remember what his doctor said about taking Viagra during treatment.

Not that it matters.

Neither one of them finish, leaving Steve to jerk off to his muted cell phone while pretending to take a shit. Even worse, Mrs. Steve crosses the finish line in the other room thinking about that bulky bald guy from the gym.

How's that for irony?

The time and money (between $20 and $80 a month) that goes into this sort of rouse hardly seems worth it, especially when you consider how the story ends. Shortly after the divorce,

Steve will run into his ex-wife and she'll be with that same bald guy from the gym. The worst part is Steve won't be able to say shit because buddy had the stones to go bald while Steve took the easy way out. He'll be forever owned by bald men.

Steve's probably living out of boxes in his new shit hole apartment, but he has hair now — *something must be going his way*. Maybe he manages to get with that new intern without getting fired? Maybe that hair restores his confidence and it pushes him over the top for a promotion?

Sure, for awhile it may seem like Steve and his hair are on the up-and-up, but don't be fooled. Balding is like death in the *Final Destination* movies, you can't escape it.

Nick Calathes thought otherwise. For years, the twenty-four year-old point guard bounced around the minor leagues before eventually finding his way to the NBA's Memphis Grizzlies. Standing 6' 6", with a chiseled jaw and high cheekbones, Calathes is a good looking guy. With his looks and lucrative career, you'd think if anyone could handle hair loss, it'd be him, right?

Wrong.

Calathes tried to run but there was nowhere to hide, and prior to the playoffs, was suspended for failing a drug test. It was surprising to say the least, since Calathes was hardly known for windmill jams or chase down blocks. He wasn't Vince Carter, jumping over seven footers, brutalizing rims across the country. What bargain bin PED was he taking?

The answer? None.

Supposedly, Calathes failed the drug test due to a steroid used in his treatment for hair loss. Labelled a cheat, he was left without a suitor in free agency and fell out of the NBA. Nowadays, he's playing in Europe with a heavy heart and a bald head.

OTHER EASY WAYS OUT

METHOD	THE SCOOP
Laser Combs	For north of $300 a month, you can lazer-comb your hair like the trek-nerd you are. There's a good chance it'll do nothing and end up in storage with your Sauna Pants and other shit you bought off the Shopping Network.
Anti-Fungal Shampoo	Works like Rogaine and looks equally embarrassing in your medicine cabinet. You had me at anti-fungal.
Saw Palmetto Extract	Herbal remedy that stops DHT production (and maybe your balls from working). But since your balls are already suspect, have at it, hoss!
Hair Cloning	By the time this is available, we'll all be under water.
Latisse	This is all unnatural, alien shit.
Hair Plugs	Don't be a bitch.

I didn't want to end up like Steve, with his aggravated scalp and wounded ego, and I didn't want to be Nick Calathes, looking over my shoulder wondering when hair loss would come and finish the job. So, I made the choice fight it clean and go without treatment.

My advice is save your money. You don't have to go medical or fly to Germany for underground treatments. Since men have been balding, they've been finding ways hide it. I'm talking the naturals. I'm talking about hats, haircuts and hair styles.

Hats

It may seem obvious, but just like hairstyles there's right and wrong ways to wear hats. Hence, the rules:

Rule #1: Be one with your hat.

If your hat's going to replace your hair it needs to be an extension of yourself. For example, if you smoke pot and wanna be the chill guy, go for the beanie (or toque, as it's known in Canada). If you want to look chill while staying on trend, the dad hat boldly states how much you care about looking like you *don't* care. You can also go dad with the rolled up toque, ditching the droopy look for something more mature. Think gritty fisherman or police informant working the loading dock.

Tough guys can opt for the toque or the flat-brimmed thug hat, but only if it's forwards or backwards. Never wear the thug hat sideways, a la *Fresh Prince*, and be sure to remove all of those shiny brim stickers. Stickers are garbage, not status symbols.

TURN *DON'T* HATS INTO *DO* HATS

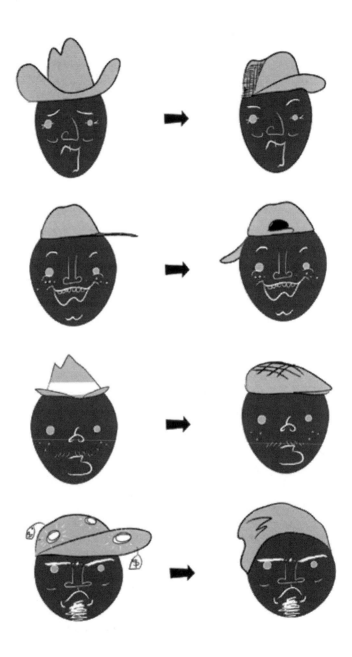

If you're from a small town and want to rep your rural roots, the trucker hat's a subtle alternative to the Stetson. It whispers, "I'm a country boy", rather than blaring it from an F-150.

Rule #2: Any hat that's key to a Halloween costume should be at the end of the bench, never part of the general rotation. *See cowboy hat.*

Rule #2 is the ceiling to Rule #1. While you should strive to find a hat that represents you, you can't let it define you. We're trying to be quiet with our hats. We're not trying to be Slash.

Rule #3: Ease into them

Hats are like the ring from *Lord of the Rings*, capable of greatness, but they can do more harm than good.

For example, There was this guy in college named Simon who had this wavy, bouncy, Sideshow Bob thing going on. People remember hair like that, so when Simon started popping up at back-to-back parties wearing a black bowler it was a little jarring. Unlike the way you'll notice someone's weight gain more when you see them infrequently, Simon drew attention to his thinning curls. The constant bowler hat was too much too soon. He should have introduced it slowly, the one-day-on, three-days-off, kind of thing. Instead, he wound up outing himself—rookie mistake—trying to be the hat guy overnight. Rule of thumb is to integrate your hats like you would a new girlfriend to your social circle, slow and steady.

As a bald man, pictures will be tough. Photo albums turn into hat museums if you aren't careful, and nothing says bald like a hat-filled gallery. Push yourself to take pictures sans hat like you push yourself to go jogging. You can have a hat photo on cheat day.

Rule #4: There's a time and place

Don't be the guy wearing a hat in the pool and don't be the chode who thinks fedoras are formalwear. Fedoras aren't any wear. Never wear them. Fedoras are for Dick Tracy and *Mad Men*, and I highly doubt you're Don Draper.

Remember Jim from high school, the guy who wrote screenplays with the most prepubescent mustache this side of the hamster cage? Jim wore a fedora. You know better.

I like to think I had the foresight not to hang my hat on hats. In the immortal words of George Costanza, "What if I meet a woman? I'd always be worried about that first moment where I'd take it off and see the look of disappointment on her face."

He's right, and I, for one, never wanted to live in fear of that inevitable day. Imagine getting ready for your first date, brushing your teeth, sculpting your beard. You're feeling pretty good, until you remember you were wearing a hat when you first met. You'll try to convince yourself she's one of these girls the blogs talk about, the kind who's under 25 and for some reason still loves Bruce Willis.

You'll try to believe it, you really will, but then you'll crumble and reach for your hat. It's your push-up bra, your Spanx. You're the ugly girl hiding behind ten pounds of makeup. You're a fraud.

A friend of mine was on a date once, rocking a beanie, when his girl launched into a story about her creepy professor.

"He used to walk around, kinda' hunched over like a dinosaur," she described. "He wore those rapist-looking glasses, and to top it off, he was bald."

"Bald? *Really*?" said my friend, tugging his toque.

"Yeah! Like, super bald. I couldn't focus in class 'cause he was, like, sooo bald."

I still don't know what makes someone "*sooo*" bald as opposed to being bald bald. Also, when the fuck did bald get creepier than rapist glasses? Given her reaction to a bald man in his forties, a bald guy in his twenties would rank straight disfigurement.

The point of wearing hats is to hide the premature balding that's almost expected for older men. However, as buddy's blind date shows, it may not matter.

Regardless, while I dabbled in hats, hair styling was more my thing. While I receded and thinned on top, I saw virtually no damage to my crown. Basically, I had a balding pattern guys would kill for.

Haircuts and Hairstyles

Haircuts become a sort of masochist ritual as you continue to lose your hair. "Not too much off the top" becomes your mantra as the scissors flash and snip, taking pieces of your childhood, your adolescence, your future with each thinning lock.

I clung to the Weber until the wheels came off, then, as my bangs continued to dissipate, developed a compensation strategy. By increasing the "wind effect" or "sweep" of my bangs, I was able to decrease the space between individual hairs for a fuller effect. Hair from above my ears was swept across my forehead for more coverage, distracting the eye with suggested motion while maintaining a solid shape. The thinner my bangs got, the higher I'd sweep them on my forehead, where they'd blend with the sweep from above my ear. This is called the *Intersection Point.*

Now, this strategy isn't for everyone. If you have dark hair and light skin it'll never work because of the high-contrast. In fact, if you have dark hair and light skin just skip this chapter and shave your head now. There's no saving you, soldier.

THE ANATOMY OF A SWEEP

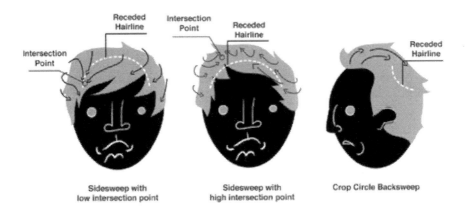

Consider this redemption for light-haired guys like me, who'll never boast 5 o'clock shadow. It's the reason my month-old mustache looks like an Italian eighth-grader's. You'll always see white skin peeking through black hair, just like you'll always see a single, black hair on white skin. It's your basic balding colour theory.

You'll also have a hard time with the sweep if your balding pattern is a two-pronged, simultaneous attack from the front and back. Sure, you'll be able mask the exposed forehead with the side-hair sweep, but that'll leave your crown vulnerable. You need to sweep towards one intersection point or else you're opening yourself up to a super weird part. The only solution is to comb the bangs over while slicking the rest back to hide the crown.

That'll look . . . *different*.

This is where things get dicey. As soon as you start saying "comb-over", your days are numbered. There's a big difference between a bald-masking hairstyle and a Donald Trump. At some point, you've gotta have the nuts to say, "It's over."

You knew about the comb-over long before you started reading *MensHairForum.com*. It's masochism. It's embarrassing. It's the guy stranded in the friend zone, giving foot rubs and listening to girl talk.

I shouldn't have to talk to you about comb-overs, but someone out there's wearing a fedora. Someone's dropping $895 on space technology called the *Theradome LH80 Pro Laser Comb*! Believe me, guys do stupid shit when they're balding, but if you're combing it over, this is bigger than hair! You need to re-evaluate your relationships because the people you're calling friends and family are lying to you. You *don't* look fine! Your haircut *doesn't* look nice! They don't respect you, they don't love you, and right now, that's what you need.

It's about to get dark, and you're gonna need support. Solid parents and siblings, friends who've faced adversity, your dog, and hopefully a girlfriend who thinks you're funny.

Hear that sound? It's the wind, threatening to mess up

your calculated disguise and literally blow your cover. You've heard it for the past few months getting louder and louder, displacing your sweep and exposing your skull. You thought you could ignore it, hoped it would go away, but deep down you knew.

No matter how much you scrunched your forehead when measuring, no matter how many virgins in the olive oil, no matter how many times you screamed, "None off the top!", you knew it was a losing battle.

Bald is coming . . . and you can't stop it.

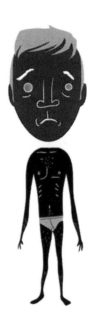

DE-FEAT-ED

adjective

"demoralized and overcome by adversity"

"Ok, Kyle, let's see."

"Gimmie a second," I say. "I want to look at it first."

I brush my head aggressively with a towel once more before unveiling the new me in the privacy of the bathroom.

I unwrap the towel from my head, releasing the lilac smell from the specialty conditioner. This must be what it feels like after a nose job, I think to myself. *What if I don't like it? What if I don't like the new me?* As though I was ever doing this for me.

I drop the white towel to the floor and confirm the transformation. I am Kyle's evil twin. I am Dark Kyle.

"Kyle!" mom shouts. "Open the door!"

I'm not ready to face her yet. The conditioner made my hair too bouncy, too formed, like I'm wearing a wig made of Jello. I turn on the faucet and quickly dunk my head for that "caught in the rain" look.

Much better.

I open the bathroom door and show my mom. Her reaction is socks on Christmas morning.

"Well," she sighs, "it's black alright . . ."

I know what she's thinking. *My son looks like 1960's Ringo Starr.* She's not totally wrong, but she's an adult, she just doesn't get it! To anyone my own age, *this* black hair with *these* jeans and this wristband turn me into some *Warped Tour* punk rocker.

Now, I don't expect you to know what that is, and frankly, it doesn't matter. What matters is *Lisa* knew what it meant, and this was all for her.

I chased after Lisa for most of grade ten, befriending her friends, helping with homework, agreeing that Chelsea was a total

40

bitch, then agreeing that Chelsea was totally bff material . . . all with minimal success.

Looking back, I can't blame Lisa for initially drawing the line at hugs and high-fives. I was a gangly ginger on the lower tier of the social ladder in that "classroom friend but lunchtime stranger" category.

This is as far as I got with my God-given attributes, but $12.99 and a few rinses later, we were slow dancing to Savage Garden at the Halloween dance. It was the classic Guy-likes-Girl, Girl-Isn't-Interested, Guy-Changes-Everything-About-Himself-to-Bend-to-Girl's-Taste story. It's timeless.

Armed with my black hair, Lisa and I made snowmen, saw movies and shared milkshakes for the next 3 years. I dyed it a few more times and experimented with a few weird cuts just to stay exciting (even rocking a two-toned thing for a while). Black hair and *The OC* were the catalysts for my high school dating life. I was the alternative semi-goth with Seth Cohen charm, emotionally-loaded for any existential conversation, quick to empathize and ready to go. Perfect for any girl looking to rebel in the safest possible way.

As it turns out, lots of teenage girls are looking for that faux rebellion and before I knew it, I had options. But despite my newfound market I remained focused on Lisa. College loomed, and we were the real deal . . .

Dystopia

It's the year 2025 and time machines sell like family sedans. Your friend's just returned from a Nirvana concert, your boss is on a stone-age vacation, and a group of activists have successfully stopped the Trump presidency. I'm packing my bags to go back to January 2007 with a bald head and a message to my younger self: Dump your girlfriend.

I close the hatch, buckle in, and flip the switch. Lights blink and needles dance. A flash of light I'm on my way.

I arrive in 2007 at 2:00 a.m. on a Friday. I grab the spare key from my parent's garage and let myself in. I creep up the stairs, hang a right down the hall, and stop at the last door on the left. I press my ear to the door and hear rustling blankets.

I creek the door open to find 17-year-old me wrapped in a grey blanket surrounded by basketball posters and dirty laundry.

"Psst, Kyle," I whisper. "It's your future self, I know you're awake."

He doesn't move.

"Kyle, seriously, I need to talk to you."

Nothing.

"Idiot," I mumble, reaching for the TV remote on the nightstand.

Immediately Kyle springs to life, jumping at the remote. He's too slow, as the TV lights the room in a flickering blue glow.

"Are you fucking serious?" I spit, watching a big-haired brunette buck back and forth in a horse-drawn carriage. "*Red Shoe Diaries*? You're watching *Red Shoe Diaries*?"

"I was sleeping!" Kyle whines, raising his hands in protest. "I swear!"

I shake my head. "So your TV just happens to be on Showcase? Name one show on Showcase that isn't *Red Shoe Diaries*."

Kyle stutters, "They...they...they play like... movies and stuff! I was watching a movie!"

"A movie?" I scoff. "Were they playing *Swordfish* again?" "You know they censor Halle Berry's boobs on TV, right?"

"It wasn't *Swordfish!*" Kyle stutters, looking around the room for an explanation. "It was...it was..."

"Dude, the volume's at zero! I know what you were doing, I'm your future fucking self."

Kyle relents, covering his lap with a pillow. "Okay, you caught me. Big deal!"

I kick some laundry to the base of the door. "If you're gonna watch this garbage at least cover the crack under your door. I could see light from the TV in the hallway."

"Shit! Seriously?" Kyle gasps.

I ignore the question, watching the brunette gaze into a foggy meadow, tracing her partner's oiled chest with her finger.

"You know there's actual porn on the internet, right?" I say. "This is like jerking off to some Harlequin novel from the grocery store."

"I can't go online!" Kyle gasps. "What if I get a virus? What if Dad goes through the Search History?"

"Dad can't even charge his Ipod," I say, slapping Kyle on the side of the head. "We've talked about this!"

43

"Fine," he grunts. "I get it, you can go now."

I shake my head. "That's not why I'm here." I take a seat on the edge of the bed. "I've got a message from the future. It's about Lisa."

Kyle comes to life again, suddenly cheering. "Yo!" he says. "I slept with her last week! We finally did it!"

"I know," I say, taking a breath. "That's why I'm here. You've got to break up with her."

Kyle starts to protest but falls silent when I hand him a photograph from my pocket: His college grad photo.

"Good Lord!" he cries. "What happened?"

"It starts during your freshman year," I explain. "By graduation you'll be over 50% bald."

Kyle stays glued to the photo. "You...you...you lied to me!" he says, brushing at his black hair. "You said you were a swimmer!"

"Kyle!"

"You said you shaved it!" he cries. "You shaved it to be aerodynamic! You wanted to reduce drag!"

"Kyle!" I interrupt. "You were just a kid! I couldn't risk telling you the truth! Who knows what you would've done! You would've been traumatized!"

"How do you think I feel now!?"

"Kyle!" I shout, "This is why I'm here! This is why you need to break up with Lisa! You need to live out your prime with nothing holding you back!"

Kyle scowls. "My prime? I lost my virginity last week! I

weigh 100 pounds, I can't even get into a bar!"

I let him vent—it's a tough pill to swallow. I remove my backpack and take out a yellow envelope marked "Motivation".

"What's this?" he asks, unfolding the top of the envelope. He holds it upside down and dumps a series of photographs onto the bed. "Who are these people?"

"Look closely," I say. "These are all girls you know. You go to school with them, they're friends of friends, you have them on MySpace, and you've got a shot with all of them."

Kyle squints at one of the images. "Is this Victoria?" he asks.

"She looks great, doesn't she? Pretty amazing what a few years can do."

"You're kidding me!" Kyle laughs, fixated on the photo. "She looks amazing!"

"In two months," I explain, "her friend will try to set you up. I rejected the idea, but you're gonna go for it. You're going to date her for two months and then you'll break up with her."

"Two months?" Kyle questions. "Why only two months?"

"You get in and you get out," I say, grabbing another photo. "Then it's on to the next one."

"But look at her! She's a rocket!"

"You don't get it 'cause you're just a kid!" I yell. "You haven't lived your twenties yet! I have to see these women on Facebook every day, knowing they *could* have been a notch in my belt! You don't know what it's like to live with this regret! I'm your future self, just listen to me!"

There's a muffled knock on the wall.

"Kyle?" Mom calls from the next room, "Is that your future self? Is everything ok?"

"Sorry mom!" I shout, knocking back. "We're cool, go back to sleep!" It's late and she works in the morning.

"Look," I say, lowering my voice. "I know you think everything's great, but you're on a dark path." I start collecting the pictures. "As it stands, you're set to date Lisa for another two years. But things change. October, 2011 you get a bad . . . let's say revealing, haircut. Lisa seems fine, even say she likes it . . . but later, you'll have a big fight about absolutely nothing. The fights will keep happening; until you part ways in the winter of 2012 . . . Your first bald year.

Kyle sits, slack-jawed, waiting for me to connect the dots.

I do.

"I've had sex with one person!" I shout. "Why do you think I know so much about internet porn?" My voice cracks. "I made a commitment and she left me, just like my hair! Now I'm bald and alone! She was all I knew! I can't even talk to cashiers!"

Kyle hands me a tissue and I turn, dabbing my eyes. "I'm so sorry," he says. "But I don't understand. How's dating keep me from going bald?"

"It doesn't," I sniff. "But if you can sleep with enough women . . . it might change the future; give me the confidence I need to look them in the eyes again. Maybe even . . . get a job, rejoin society . . ."

Kyle looks like he might be sick. "I . . . I don't know," he manages.

"Ten women," I say. "That's all I ask. Ten women over the

next three years. I think double digits'll really do a lot for . . . uh, us."

I wipe my nose, the TV's glow reflecting in my watery eyes. Kyle pats me on the back and says he'll do his best. I thank him and turn for the door.

"Hey, future self," he says.

I stop. "Yeah?"

"The Raptors just drafted Andrea Bargnani. Is he really gonna be the next Dirk Nowitzki?"

So young, so innocent.

I take a deep breath and survey my childhood bedroom one last time.

"No," I exhale. "He isn't."

*****

No one expects their prime to come and go by eighteen because no teenager expects to get hit with male pattern baldness. I was the '91 Chicago Bulls fresh off an NBA championship—I didn't expect Jordan to go play baseball in '93.

At twenty-one, I gave up on olive oil, the infrequent washes, the frequent washes, and all the other half-baked hair schemes I'd become a slave to. I looked in the mirror, recalling the first time I dyed my hair despite being told it increased hair loss. I remembered all the times I'd made fun of my dad or poked fun at guys with comb-overs. It gave me an eerie, karmic feeling, like my carelessness or insensitivity had caused this to happen.

I was the guy in Titanic who scoffs "The ship can't sink!"

only to try sneaking on a lifeboat moments later, blending in with women and children like a coward. I think part of me loves that movie because I empathize with the characters. That sinking feeling they get when the iceberg hits—*I've lived it.* I felt that same certainty of doom, knowing it's only a matter of time before I'm sunk.

In the last chapter I discussed a few ways I tried to stay on the ship or sneak onto a lifeboat, but we're past that now. The lifeboats have left. The ship is at 10 o'clock and the band has stopped playing. Remember when you were king of the world?

At times it felt like the sinking feeling was an actual symptom of becoming less attractive. Just like staring at a computer screen can cause headaches, my depression and general malaise was the byproduct of becoming an ugly person. I was transforming. I was devolving.

As men we often throw jabs at women for their insecurity. We laugh when they ask if they look fat in their jeans and scoff at the endless hours they spend applying makeup. But the truth is, we're just as insecure.

When hair loss hits, you too will start obsessing over your appearance. You'll be totally chicked-out, wondering how others see you.

We all know the girl who fixates on her stretch marks or that bulge around her waistline. She spends her weekends binging *Friends* on DVD, eating Nutella from the jar—*it's not chocolate, it's hazlenut spread*! She thinks shopping vigorously counts as exercise, yet she complains about her "pudge" and it drives you crazy. You want to shake her! Her ass should look like a topographical map by now! If you can't stand the heat, get out of the kitchen—don't *eat* the kitchen! She should have seen this coming and handled her shit long ago!

To that, I can relate.

I'm built like a coat hanger with a Usain Bolt metabolism. I think gyms are for meatheads and have actually argued that standing's a workout because I'm supporting my own weight, making every day leg day. As the artsy guy, I could get away with it because being skinny played to my strengths. Take away my hair, though, and I'm a cancer patient, a fucking candy apple.

When balding hit, I suddenly looked at my body with a sense of shock. Like, when the fuck did this happen? Why don't I have muscles? I'm twenty-one going on thirteen! Like the fat girl shot-gunning ketchup, I completely blanked on cause and effect.

"Why'd you let me quit swimming?" I bitched to my parents. "Have you seen Michael Phelps and that V-taper? That could have been me!"

It felt like hair was the only thing that kept me presentable. If time machines really were a thing, I'd tell my younger self to hit the weights and slam some egg whites. If he complained I'd say, "Scroll though *#mancrushmonday* on Instagram and stop when you find a skinny, bald man."

#handcramp.

With my appearance in a toilet-like tailspin, it was only a matter of time before I discovered my feminine side. We've all dated the girl who talks about her future husband right out of the gate. She's only interested in your career ceiling and asks questions that gauge your ability to be a good father.

Balding did that to me, too.

Joan was a girl I knew on Facebook. She was relatively attractive with a good head on her shoulders and a seemingly positive trajectory. After a few conversations online, I casually

49

slipped in a not-so-subtle, "So, how do you feel about bald men?"

"I dunno," she replied. "I like that guy from *Crank*."

Was Joan interesting? *No.* Was she fun? *No.* Did she give me butterflies or make me nervous? Not at all, but she liked the guy from *Crank,* and when your hairline's waning, you've gotta lock that shit up.

To me, Joan became wifey material.

First date, I took her to my work Christmas party and introduced her to my parents. That might seem forward, but I was on a timeline. Regardless, I don't remember much about the night except for being totally pissed I didn't get a second date. I didn't care that she rejected me—I didn't even like her—I was pissed because she fucked up my plan. She was supposed to marry me to mask the fact that balding would turn me into an undateable creature. She was supposed to marry me so I could hide from my insecurities. People would say, "Well, he got her. I must be missing something."

Goddammit Joan! Why couldn't you just buy in!?

Needless to say, I realized I wasn't going to find a wife all that quickly. I needed to change my draft strategy.

The Experiment

Let me preface this by saying male pattern baldness is no joke. My insecurities were at an all-time high and concern for my appearance began to dominate my psyche. Eventually, painfully, I came to accept I'd look like an alien the rest of my life. I was going bald and that wasn't going to change, but maybe I could change my taste in women.

I studied a year of psychology at University of Toronto and finished with a solid 67% thanks to a cushy multiple choice exam. I attended just over half of my classes and jotted notes like, "*Psychoanalysis—that episode of Ren and Stimpy with the horse*". In other words, you could deem me as somewhat knowledgeable of the mind.

One thing I do remember is Pavlov's dogs.

Basically, some guy named Pavlov couldn't feed his dogs until late at night because he worked as a bartender or something. Anyways, he noticed his starving dogs start slobbering whenever they heard his keys in the front door because they came to expect food when he got home.

There's ways we've all been conditioned just like Pavlov's dogs. For example, I get queasy at the sight of green sponges because they trigger a bad experience with KFC coleslaw. I can't hear the words "little by little" without singing it back because of that song by Oasis.

I was running out of options and getting pretty comfortable at rock bottom when I had this desperate idea: maybe somehow, some way, I could condition myself to be attracted to conventionally unattractive women.

Hmmm.

I figured by the time I was totally bald I'd be hideous, so when I say unattractive, I don't mean big nose, broad shoulders, bad teeth, etc. I'm talking years of drug abuse, Yak-women, sideshow shit. I remembered my mom taping a photo of four enormous women on the fridge as motivation to eat healthier. That's what I was going for, the '*I'm-gonna-change-my-ways-so-I-don't-end-up-looking-like-her*' look.

I wondered: What would happen if I started a masturbation regimen to pictures of attractive women, then, at the moment of orgasm, flipped to photos from *Faces of Meth* or the cast of *The View*? Could I eventually create a subconscious association between sexual release and these sorts of women? Could I bend my brain into creating an ugly fetish?

I thought I could.

Was it really that crazy?

Yes. Yes it was.

The real question is why would I want an ugly fetish? Well, obviously I *wouldn't*, but I didn't want to be bald. I didn't want to look like a skeleton, and I didn't want to spend my life pining for women who'd never give me a shot.

In other words, I was terrified I'd never find a fulfilling relationship. What if the woman I fell in love with couldn't get past my big, bald head?

I once spoke to a financial therapist, someone who specialized in things like overspending, penny-pinching, or general financial obsessions. She said many of her patients were multi-millionaires who called in the middle of the night with panic attacks over thoughts of losing their wealth.

I bring this up in relation to vanity. I don't think their fear was simply going broke, but rather, going broke while maintaining the expensive tastes they'd become accustomed to. It's not about the money, but the lifestyle that came with it.

I was never hung up on my appearance until I thought I'd wake up looking like an earthworm, out of the running with the types of women I'd grown used to. The idea, therefore, was to psycho-fuck my brain into feeling attracted to anyone who'd give me the time of day—anyone as desperate as me—so I could not only survive the transition from filet to fish sticks . . . but be happy with it.

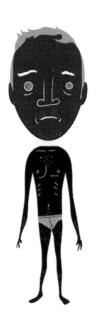

AC-CEPT-ANCE

noun

"willingness to tolerate a difficult or unpleasant situation"

Although I still think it has legs, I never actually conducted my experiment and neither should you. As with any psychosexual tinkering, you can't help but consider the side effects: random erections in public places, orgasms every time you come across *The View*. It's the sort of thing that results in those guys who fall in love with their cars or drool over stuffed animals. Regardless, it was a total pipe dream. No amount of conditioning was gonna make me okay with going bald.

Maybe you can relate or maybe my nightmare was a little darker than yours. Maybe your hair loss is just one in a series of aging symptoms, the cherry on top of your glasses-wearing, nose-hair-plucking, crows-feet-mess-of-a-head and I didn't realize how lucky I was?

Regardless, I didn't feel lucky. At twenty-two I accepted my fate. This would be my life. . .

My Bald Life

I wake around 8:20, pretty late considering I start work at 9. But it's no problem. See, I'm bald so no one notices I've prioritized sleep over showers for the last five days.

Outside, I shiver in the cold waiting for the bus. The Canadian winters are worse than ever without hair sealing in the heat. Even with a hat, I miss the layer of insulation my hair used to provide. I really miss it when the sleet turns my hat into a cold, damp washcloth, keeping my head wet and clammy, adding to my misery.

No one sits beside me on the bus. I used to think I'd like

that but now it bothers me. Am I that off-putting? Maybe it's because my soggy hat and poor hygiene leave me in a constant state of sickness? Or maybe it's the resting bitch-face I've developed after years of feeling inadequate.

Regardless, I slog to work and head for my cubicle. I work a shitty office job—thanks, Liberal Arts degree—staring at spread sheets all day. Over time this sort of work has left me near-sighted, peering through glasses with the least dweeby frames I could find. I don't socialize much because I've creeped out all the girls, making me a virus to all the guys looking to score. As a result, I often get sidetracked by all the online dating profiles I've made—*Plenty of Fish, OKCupid, LavaLife*—featuring photos of me cropped at the forehead. However, my inbox reads zero and my calendar's empty.

Maybe I'll buy a fedora.

My measure of success in life comes from a list of check boxes tied to things like *House, Girlfriend, Good Job*, etc. It's not a literal list, just an ongoing tally in my head. Right now, the only thing checked is *Family*, the clan sticking with me through thick and . . . well, you know.

I unchecked the *Friends* box some time ago as most of them got into relationships or simply stopped returning my texts. I went from being a key group member to being the guy who occupied the ugly girl while our friends mingled. Eventually I couldn't even fill that role and was cut from the team. Maybe I should rethink the whole shower thing . . .

Regardless, my deteriorating social life leads to little action on Facebook and Twitter. I just sort of scroll, and scroll, and scroll . . .

By now, I think I've made myself clear: balding sucks, blah, blah, blah. Are you sick of it yet? Do you think I'm trying to pad the page count? If you're in the same boat, you've probably dragged on with similar dredging to anyone who'll listen. Why do you keep talking about it? Why can't you let go? It's over!

Well, not for everyone.

At twenty three, I *could* let it go, but others couldn't. Clearly, I was going bald—my bangs were a mess of tumbleweeds starting half way up my skull. Why was it so hard for others to confirm the obvious: "Yes Kyle, you *are* going bald."

To answer that question, let's revisit the girlfriend who keeps harassing you about her fat jeans. You tell her she looks fine, but she keeps hounding you. Same question, same jeans, same fat ass. You say, "Babe, look at you! You're being ridiculous!" like you're some kind of smooth-talking casanova. Meanwhile, she's a mess of insecurity because you keep avoiding the truth.

Ever wonder if she knows she looks fat? Maybe she isn't looking for compliments but rather some sort of assurance that despite her weight she's still attractive. In my case, I wasn't looking for the "Don't be silly, you're fine!" support, I was looking for the, "Your ass is huge and I love it!" support.

Imagine if a friend came out of the closet and your response was, "Nah, you're just a little eccentric." In this hyper-sensitive age, you'd be crucified! What I'm saying is there's nothing wrong with being gay, nothing wrong with love handles, and nothing wrong with going bald.

That's what I needed to hear.

Instead, my parents would say, "You've got a full head of hair, you just need to mess it up!" My friends were no better, saying, "Your hair's always looked like that." Even Nick—the asshole who started the whole thing—backed off, "A joke," he shrugged. "To get under your skin.

Really.

I imagined them holding secret meetings, coming up with ways to keep me from the truth like Jim Carey in *The Truman Show*. Photoshopping old photos while I slept, thinning their own hair to make mine seem normal. It's a conspiracy!

Just the thought of it made me so anxious I needed to make sure everyone knew *I knew* I was balding. It felt like strangers on the street were whispering, "That hat isn't fooling anyone," like I was some kind of joke. We laugh at the mouth-breathers passed out on the subway, snot dripping down their faces, all boogery and stupid, yet don't laugh at the cold-sufferers—tissues in hand, nose dripping, eyes leaky—'cause they know they're a mess. *They're in on the joke.*

I wanted to shout from a mountaintop, send out a mass email: "I'm Kyle and I'm going bald! I know it, you know it! I've struggled with it, and now I'm accepting it."

I got to the point where I'd obsessed over my hair loss for four years and was sick of obsessing. I'd been fighting to keep my hair, begging it to stay: "Baby, I'll change! I'll throw away my hats! I won't dye you anymore! I swear!"

It was time I stood up for myself and said what I was really feeling: "Hair, I don't know what happened, but you've turned into a total bitch and I can't take it anymore. I'd take the high road but lost the will to be a gentleman a long fucking time ago. That new look you're rocking is a disaster and everyone's laughing at you, including me. It's over!"

Shaving My Head

It's fitting that I end my story where it began: in front of the bathroom mirror. "Well, here we are," I say to my reflection, seemingly for the last time.

I don't speak aloud (I may be balding but I'm not crazy). I don't need to. My reflection's been with me every step of the way. He knows my, "What are they talking about?" smirks, my half-hearted looks of feigned confidence, my gaunt, worrisome stares.

He knows this is it.

Game time.

Choosing between the buzzer and razor is like choosing between the electric chair and lethal injection. One's loud and dramatic, the other sleek and silent, but both'll get you to the same place. I opt for the buzzer, scared that shaving too close to the skin will leave ingrown hairs or pimples like shaving my face sometimes does. Being bald with Freddy Kruger skin is the last thing I need.

I take off my shirt to keep it from getting hairy. My skin's ghostly white and my body skeleton thin, only fitting I cap it off with a matching skull.

I flip the power button and the buzzer starts to hum. The humming turns to a low growl, drowning me in white noise as it moves closer and closer to my ear.

I give one last goodbye to my reflection, and take in one of the rare and authentic "first day of the rest of my life" moments before turning the blade on myself.

I run a strip front to back above my right ear followed by another strip beside it, buzzing my head the same way I'd mow the lawn, row by row until there's nothing left.

Red whiskers, sprinkling dandruff, and other debris rain onto my shoulders and chest while tufts collect on the bathroom floor. Other refugees find shelter behind the faucet and on the mirror's ledge, huddling together until the genocide is over and the transformation is complete.

There's no grand unveiling like the day I dyed my hair black. Like the difference between takeoff and landing, this wasn't thrilling or exciting, more a tired sigh of relief.

I stand in the bathroom, naked and bald as the day I was born. I brush my head over the trash bin before looking in the mirror with a sense of accomplishment. Then I have it, my first bald breakthrough: *Being* bald looks better than *going* bald.

Without my hairline drawing attention, my once-giant forehead seems to shrink to a proportionate size. My head looks smaller, making my shoulders seem broader and my skeletal body a little less skeletal.

Last year's brush cut didn't mislead me. The shape of my skull is second to none, and the blemishes I was so afraid of are nowhere to be found.

Shaving my head feels like winning a board game I'd been losing. Imagine sitting with a rack of vowels while your dad plays his third "S", opening another Triple Word Score for your sister. You trade your letters just to get two more "U's" and three "I's" and without warning, smash the board. Letters fall to the

61

floor and you stomp from the table, stressed and fuming. Within minutes though, you're outside, sipping beer in the sun and it's like *Scrabble* never happened.

That's shaving your head.

The relief is overwhelming. You found your wallet! Your keys were in your other pants. You wake from the nightmare. Nothing's lost, stolen or harmed.

I'm not saying I'd trade my teen flow for this new look, but clearly, holding onto my fleeting hair wasn't doing me any favors. In fact, it's apparent how stupid I looked and how much my receding hairline was aging me. Never in my wildest dreams did I think shaving my head would actually make me look younger.

While the hair-on-the-sides, fluff-on-the-top look gets associated with old men, a clean shave seems athletic and strong. Maybe it's the military connection? Whatever the reason, it just works.

Remember Joan? The girl who liked Jason Statham in *Crank*? How do you think she'd feel if he traded his shaved head for the Friar Tuck? Suddenly he's looking a lot more like Ted from accounting than *The Transporter*. What about the Michael Jordan Jumpman? Think it would have the same effect with a few Homer Simpson tassels blowing in the wind? We can play this game all day and the answer won't change: bald is better than balding, and if you're still clinging to scraps, every passing minute is a minute lost.

Maybe I'm being too positive too fast. Maybe you're sitting there thinking, "I don't look anything like Jason Statham. This doesn't apply to me."

Believe me, I've been there: massaging oil into my scalp, reading blogs about women who love bald guys like Bruce Willis, feeling hopeless because I'm totally *not* Bruce Willis.

But then I came to realize that no one is Bruce Willis. *Not even Bruce Willis.*

Strip away his *Die Hard* characters and put him in a grey hoody doing physio at the Y. Take away his gun and throw him in the produce isle sporting a smock at minimum wage. Our perception of Bruce Willis is rooted in the characters he portrays— women don't love Bruce Willis, they love Harry Stamper and John McClane—not because of their looks, but because they bust skulls and kick ass.

Look at whatever fraying nest you have left and ask yourself, is that the hair of someone who kicks ass? How many action figures sell with that hair? How many first-person-shooters have Johnny Rogaine looking down the barrel? Do you wanna be Schwarzenegger's "Mr. Freeze" or Divito's "Penguin"?

It's time to be a man and kick some ass.

It's time to shave your head.

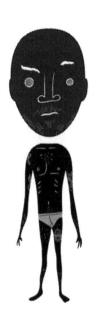

A-DAPT

verb

"become adjusted to new conditions"

The Dream

"I had the dream again."

Kelly rolls over and tucks her head under my arm. I lay on my back, eyes on the blank ceiling, trying to hold onto the feeling.

"Yeah?" Kelly moans, disinterested, barely awake.

"It was the same as last time," I say. "But different . . . like, the same scene but . . ."

I run my hand down the back of my head. It's the same feeling of sandpaper. Nothing's changed.

"I'm still sleeping," Kelly whines.

"It was the same scene," I continue. "I'm alone in the bathroom looking in the mirror. My hair's grown out a little, like before I buzz it . . ."

"Okay . . ." Kelly moans.

"I'm looking in the mirror, analyzing my head, combing through with my fingers. I'm about to shave, then somehow, some way, I'm able to sweep back some hair and tie it in a bun.

Kelly pauses, missing something. "I thought you said this dream was different?"

I reach for the ceiling, like the dream's floating away.

"It was. Last time, it was the whole head but this time it was just the top. I had a top knot."

I run my fingers again to the same feeling of sandpaper.

Nothing's changed.

*****

I've had the dream four times since shaving my head. Each time, I'm in the same washroom looking in the same mirror above the sink and my hair is the way it was before I first buzzed it. Each dream ends with me discovering a new way to tie my hair into a bun, and each dream leaves me equally lost.

I don't know if "lost" is the right word. It's this foggy feeling, like the guy in the dream is a version of myself living in an alternate reality, and for a few minutes my consciousness crossed over.

It feels like a memory, like my hair is a phantom limb. There's no part where I say, "Okay Kyle, you're dreaming," like the time I hung out with the Muppets and slow danced with Uma Thurman inside a snow globe. That's what makes this one so deflating. It seems so possible, like, if I just grew my hair and parted it a certain way . . .

Stop!

Walk it back . . .

I am Odysseus, tempted by the Sirens' song. Every bald man questions if he gave in too soon. You come across old photos where your sweep had good coverage, you see a few guys still hanging in there . . .

Yeah! I still have my electric guitar up in the attic! Let's get the band back together and give it one last try!

That's how you get bands like Velvet Revolver—a group nobody wanted, made of rockers no one was missing—forcing their frail, coked-up limbs into skinny leather pants, taking the stage like edgy, old lesbian women. It's how legacies are ruined and icons shattered. You went out on top. Don't be Velvet

Revolver and don't let anyone talk you into a victory lap.

Not even your subconscious.

Let's say your stubble grows fast and seems thicker than you recall. Maybe you'll take to Google and convince yourself that your follicles were clogged or dried up. Maybe they were irritated and now that your scalp's had a chance to breathe your follicles are back to normal?

That sounds like a thing! Right?

As you let it grow, you'll start to see a definite horseshoe shape where certain areas have more density than others. You'll convince yourself that the longer the hairs grow the more coverage you'll have and you'll be able to hide the horseshoe.

You're not totally wrong, but it's impossible to sweep hairs that grow up and out like porcupine quills. You'll spend months in the spikey stage before you can start sweeping your hair again. Do you really think you have the stomach for that?

I didn't think so.

I went online to find an interpretation of my bun dream. Seems the internet is loaded with bald dreams, just none about a bald man discovering he still has hair. For example:

1) Dreaming of losing your hair may mean you're stressed about the idea of getting older. It can represent a lack of spiritual protection or a warning about poor health.

2) Dreaming you're going bald can be due to a lack of self-esteem and the feeling of being unattractive.

3) Dreaming of being bald may be a warning of impending financial loss or represent the belief that you're incapable.

4) If everyone in the dream is bald except for you, it means

you're less pure than others.

5) If you dream of a bald head during a full moon, be prepared for sudden loss.

6) If you dream of bald women, it means you're in a relationship with a quarrelsome woman who may ruin your life.

7) If a woman dreams of a bald stranger, it means she should be more selective in choosing a partner.

8) If your entire dream consists of bald men, it's a sign of good weather in the next three days.

Well then . . .

Good thing I dreamt of having hair, especially since I hadn't booked a trip in the next few days. Sorry if you're having sex dreams about *V for Vendetta's* Natalie Portman, apparently your girlfriend's a bitch!

My favorite's the one about low self-esteem and the overall feeling of being unattractive. *Well, no shit!* Was I sleeping for the past five years? That's exactly how I felt!

I came up with my own interpretation, that my dream was the result of never having long hair. Not that I really wanted it, it's just that I regret not growing it while I could. I did have one of those greaser mullets for Halloween once (I went as a child predator). I liked how it felt, slicked back behind my ears and the way it curled at the back when I wore a hat. I've always regretted cutting it right after Halloween because I could almost tie it back. I never grew it that long again—I was never able to—and now I'll never know how it would have felt to tie that knot.

If you're reading this book, you probably missed the boat too. That's okay, 'cause there's a lesson to be learned. Call it *The Bald Parable*. Grow your hair while you still can because you'll never know when it'll stop growing. In other words, make the most of opportunities that come your way.

They may never come again.

Afterglow

As happy as I was to not have any weird birthmarks or bulges on my naked dome, eventually the high wore off. When it did, I came to terms with my transformation.

Now and forever, I would be a bald man.

It's a scary thought. No more hairstyles or gels to hide behind. No cuts to look older, or younger, or cooler, or smarter. I was naked, forever exposed by what was given and now taken away.

I looked in the mirror. While my shaved head looked better than I'd imagined, I was still a skinny bald guy. Nothing like Bruce Willis.

If shaving your head's like a rebirth, the next step would be growing into the person you're meant to become. When you're an infant, your development is largely dictated by your parents and the influence of other snot-nosed kids. But with your bald rebirth, you're in the driver's seat. You've established perspective and critical awareness. You can use these things to strategize your development and choose the type of bald man you'll become.

To do this, I had to take an honest look myself. I had to recognize my strengths and weaknesses, and compare them to men who were thriving without hair.

Imagine you're the parent to a 6' 5" twelve-year-old. Do you encourage them to play golf or basketball? Now, try using the same logic on yourself. What positive qualities or talents do you have that can lend themselves to your new, bald persona?

Know what? It's easier if I show you.

THE SUCCESSFUL GUY

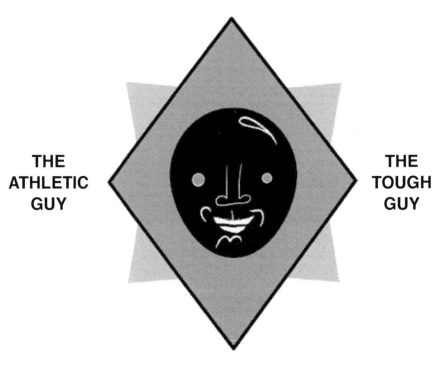

THE ATHLETIC GUY

THE TOUGH GUY

THE SPIRITUAL GUY

The Bald Persona Spectrum (BPS)

Don't get it twisted, this isn't your dad's guide to going bald. I'm not going to tell you to grow some shit beard and everything will be fine. Anyone can watch *Breaking Bad* and deduce that Walter looks way cooler with a goatee. Then what? This is the deep dive. This is character development.

On the surface you can look at bald men and see the clear divide between the Vin Diesel's and the Moby's. I came up with the BPS as a way to go beyond this, to actually define the winning characteristics of bald guys who thrive. Accordingly, I read articles and blogs, studied photos and movies to expose myself to all manner of bald. I'd be on my way to work and see a bald guy with a good-looking girl and ask myself, "What's he doing differently from the bald guy ogling from afar? What's he wearing? How's he carrying himself? What's the secret?"

My conclusion was, on the surface, most thriving bald men identified with at least one of four BPS categories: Successful Guy, Athletic Guy, Spiritual Guy, Tough Guy. I further determined that those not falling within the BPS unfortunately landed in the GWP— the *Guess Who?* Paradigm—but more on that later.

For now, let's study the four corners of the BPS, providing you with the shovel you'll need to dig yourself out of your bald hole.

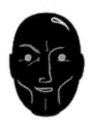

LEX LUTHOR: THE SUCCESSFUL BALD GUY

Straight out of the DC universe, Lex Luthor is a power-mad American billionaire, businessman, inventor, philanthropist and the world's smartest man. Despite his brainpower, he's overflowing with charisma and is a well-known public figure. Oh, he's also hellbent on killing Superman.

You can't compete with this. I don't care if you're rocking the trendiest man-bun in SoCal, when Lex pulls up in his drop-top Bugatti he's taking your girl and that's it. I mean, the guy fucks with Superman! He doesn't even see you.

Now, while it's unrealistic to achieve Lex Luthor's level of success—he became President for Christ sake—you *can* aspire to be *like* him. In short, with a big dick, big ego, and big paycheck you too can be the Successful Guy.

Any SBG is the product of extreme confidence and second-to-none ambition expressed through luxury. Hair? Fuck hair! You're cooking that lean shit! Closing deals and opening legs. Balding can't stop you because nothing can. You're the man.

Unfortunately, if you're flipping burgers or punching numbers into a cash register, you've got work to do. The SBG wears suits that cost more than your rent and lords the corner office with the view. Conversely, my old boss makes a shitload of money but rides the brake of his Chrysler sedan in his browned, New Balance sneakers. He's hardly Kevin O'Leary, saying things like, "The customer's always right" and "Lovely" while punching code all day.

In short, he isn't Lex Luthor. He's Clark Kent. He's got the money but lacks the swag. He needs that *Mad Men* suit and all the single malt scotch and strippers that come with it. He needs to project success. Sizzle and steak.

Now, while I'm good with money, Successful Guy isn't my play. I'm t-shirts and jeans with glasses perched on my nose like some old librarian. Not only that, I went to art school. It's pretty hard to exude wealth and possession-fueled confidence zipping through traffic like the Great Gazoo on a Craigslist bike.

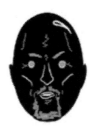

STONE COLD: THE TOUGH BALD GUY

Sure, wrestling is ballet for dudes, and waxed chests aren't exactly the image of barbaric masculinity, but Stone Cold Steve Austin is pure testosterone. He's steak marinated in diesel fuel, a pit bull giving the finger. Say otherwise and there's a Stone Cold Stunner with your name on it.

Stone Cold is the spirit of every biker gang and bouncer. Rocking a leather vest and bluejeans, he's a broad, beer-drinking, redneck too irrational to solve problems with words. Standing at 6'2 and 270 pounds, he's the face of the WWE's Attitude Era, and the epitome of bald toughness.

The Tough Bald Guy image is tried and true. Maybe it's a prison thing or a result of soldiers buzzing down. Maybe you just don't notice a guy's haircut when he's got traps to his ears? Whatever the reason, the badder you are, the balder you can be. It's nature.

Along with his brash catchphrases, Stone Cold brings something else to the tough guy table. I'm talking, of course, about facial hair.

Harken back to the bare knuckle boxers of the 1880's, twizzling handlebar mustaches with bloody digits between bouts.

Or the Vikings, beards flowing, while they pillaged and plundered with impunity. Throughout history, facial hair's exuded masculinity and toughness. As any bald man will tell you, your balls swing a bit heavier with a beard keeping your face warm. It's like some Daredevil blind shit: lose your hair and it strengthens your beard. It's a surefire way to look tough.

Now, before you declare yourself the Bald Tough Guy, you need to ask yourself, "Am I big . . . or just fat?" Be honest. Don't suck in the gut or hide under giant sweaters. Look your tits in the eye and face facts. Fat guys playing tough is an epidemic. Every generation has at least one fat rapper who pretends to be a boss. Fat Joe, Rick Ross . . . does anyone take them seriously? They've got the tats and the gangster shit, but has it ever felt genuine? How do they make it through shows without dying? Do they sit on stage? There's nothing tough about sleep apnea and there's nothing badass about sweating during breakfast. If you can't take the stairs you're more than a few miles on the elliptical from being tough. You're not a mob boss, you're the fat kid in gym.

At this point I don't need to tell you that my basketball jerseys hangs in a shadowbox for a reason. Shoulders like mine were meant to be clothed. In other words, I'm more than a few chicken breasts from being the Tough Bald Guy.

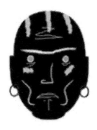

DHALSIM: THE SPIRITUAL BALD GUY

We go from one fighter to the next.

In the heyday of *Sega* and *Super Nintendo*, Dhalsim was a character in *Street Fighter II*, the gold standard of button-mashing fighter games. Now, for anyone like me who sucked at this sort of thing, Dhalsim was the man. He had the ability to stretch his limbs so you could just chill on your side of the screen and keep your distance. He also had the Zen-fueled ability to teleport, float and breath fireballs . . . cuz, you know, yoga and stuff . . .

That's ultimately the secret for being the Spiritual Guy. Dhalsim, with his head tattoos, pierced ears, blank white eyes and necklace of shrunken skulls, mixes equal parts spirituality with mysterious badassery. Why the face tats? *Buddhism.* Missing pupils? *Hinduism.* Necklace of shrunken heads? Uh . . . *Satanism?* Who cares, it's *badass*!

With his washboard ribs, Dhalsim's probably vegan, but he gives off the cryptic vibe he could kick your ass regardless. This is important because without it, he's Ghandi; no different from the bald hippies eating granola at peaceful protests.

Dhalsim doesn't want to enlighten you, he doesn't even want to smile. He wants to be left alone to make paintings you don't understand.

Spirituality is defined as "a sense of connection to something bigger than ourselves," and doesn't necessarily involve religion. In the case of the Spiritual Guy, it's about an abstract state of mind that relieves all insecurity and social pressure. Dhalsim has an aura that suggests he didn't go bald one hair at a time like Stone Cold or Lex Luthor, but by some spiritual awakening in a flash of divine light.

I can't tell you how to be the Spiritual Guy 'cause the Spiritual guy just *is*. He makes you feel silly watching sports, saying things like, "None of this matters; it's a bunch of grown men chasing a ball." You know nothing about his job, except that it's probably cooler and more fulfilling than anything you've ever experienced.

I once saw a bald magician on *America's Got Talent* swallowing swords and shit. He was average height, average build, with a flat, wide face; nothing *GQ* about him. But just watching him address the audience you knew the guy had groupies camped outside his dressing room.

That's the Spiritual Bald Guy.

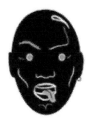

MICHAEL JORDAN: THE BALD ATHLETE

Michael Jeffery Jordan, who else would it be?

NBA champ, league MVP, All-Star, and unofficial bald ambassador. I don't need to insult His Airness with an explanation of what makes him the Athletic Guy, he's Michael fucking Jordan. Instead, I'm going to take the next few paragraphs to compare him and the so-called heir to the throne, Lebron James.

All too often, the number one guy is put on a pedestal he can't be knocked from, no matter how the competition stacks up. Like, how long are we gonna pretend Jimmy Hendrix is the best guitar player ever? Hell, some nine-year-old's already shredding *Purple Haze* off-handed on Youtube. Is that really GOAT shit?

Recently, Lebron's Cleveland Cavaliers overcame a 3-1 deficit against the best team in history to take the NBA title. Every year, he's a shoe-in for the finals, an MVP front-runner and a defensive beast. What else does he have to do? What else is there to do?

For me, it's simple. He has to shave his head.

We all saw it: sporadic hairs eroding in the corners of his forehead after a few years in the league. Then, his headbands started getting thicker, angled further and further back until one day, they vanished, suddenly replaced by a fuller head of hair.

Did he really think we wouldn't notice?

It's not like he's unaware. He's heard the jokes. He's read the comment section. He knows he's balding. Worse yet, he knows we know he knows!

Maybe that's why he joined Miami in the first place and the reason he bailed when Wade and Bosh got old. After hair loss, he needed something easy.

And that's why he'll never be Michael. Jordan didn't care about anything but winning. He didn't need to be liked, didn't need to be trendy. He needed to be the best, and everything else would follow.

Lebron, on the other hand, at 6' 8", 250, with the agility of a squirrel and the strength of a fucking rhino, puts image above all else. So much so that despite his muscles and money, his chalk-throwing and chest pounding, the "King" can't live without his fuzzy crown . . . something a schlubb like me does every goddamn day.

How's that for guts? The guy plays in the NBA, a league full of bald men—literally the safest space to lose your hair—and still remains closeted. Meanwhile, I've got the stones to overcome something one of the world's biggest celebrities can't handle.

Michael didn't wear a headband or opt for plugs, and he didn't spray his head with that weird hair-in-a-can (shout out to Carlos Boozer). Nope, Jordan shaved his head in the hyper-competitive way you'd expect him to. If he was gonna be bald he'd be the most bald. Think your scalp's shiny? *His* was shinier. Think your head's smooth? *His* was smoother. He looked in the mirror and said, "I'm Michael fucking Jordan", stuck out his tongue and handled his shit. He probably burned off his follicles with a damn laser.

81

Jordan blazed the trail and created a safe haven for anyone hiding under a hat, just in time for LeBitch to blow it up, telling you to run from adversity, to be embarrassed by what you see in the mirror.

Compare their basketball resumes and it's a toss-up, but compare them as men, as role models, and it's a Jordan clean sweep.

Hair doesn't measure heart.

*****

Successful Guy, Tough Guy, Spiritual Guy, Athletic Guy: so concludes the Bald Persona Spectrum, defining the pillars of thriving bald men.

Relating to one of the four corners is the first step in freeing you from the shackles of hair loss. If you don't land on the BPS right away, it's something to aspire to. That being said, you may have your work cut out for you, especially if you find yourself on the *Guess Who?* Paradigm—the other side of the coin.

SAM

TOM

BILL

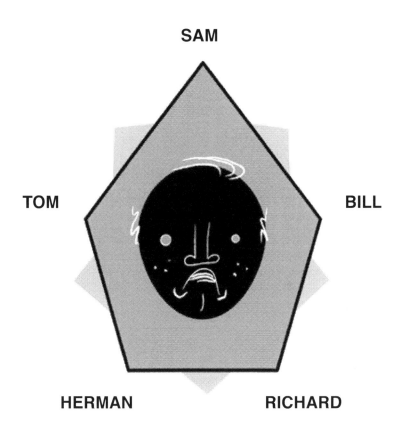

HERMAN

RICHARD

The *Guess Who?* Paradigm

The antithesis of the Bald Persona Spectrum is the *Guess Who?* Paradigm, named after 90's board game, *Guess Who?*. After choosing a character, the point of the game was to guess your opponent's character based on a series of features like glasses, hats, hair . . . or a lack thereof.

There are 5 bald guys in the game—Sam, Richard, Tom, Bill, and Herman—and just like the Bald Persona Spectrum, each character represents a corner of the GWP. While the BPS involves positive traits, this cast of failures represent the negative; the kind of men who fall victim to hair loss. You can find them alone at movie theatres or in their parent's basement all scoliosis in front of rigged computers. Defined by baldness, these men curled up in balls and let hair loss win. These are the guys you *don't* want to be.

SAM: THE BALD OLD GUY

Sam had to be included because he's a bald guy in *Guess Who?*. In reality, though, Sam's just old, and there's no shame in being bald when you're old. So, enjoy your sunrise Cracker Barrel. Hair or no hair, no one's judging you!

In other words, if you're counting white hairs on your pillow each morning you're Sam, and its fine to be Sam. Remember, this is a book about the horrors of premature baldness. There are few silver foxes in *Guess Who?* Not everyone can be as lucky as that fucker Paul.

Age happens. You have bigger things to worry about.

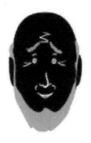

RICHARD: THE BALD PUSSY

In *Guess Who?* there are safe questions that quickly narrow the field by casting a wide net. Questions like, "Are you a woman?" or "Do you have glasses?" Alternatively, there are questions like, "Do you have a really big nose?" or "Do you wear a hat?" that are bigger gambles since they apply to fewer characters.

Now, if you were to guess, "Are you a total pussy who's dying for acceptance and approval?" you'd be swinging for the fences on Richard.

Richard is a brown-bearded bald man who looks like he was born in a tan turtleneck. He plays open-chord Christian songs and makes his own dip; not for chips or nachos, but for crackers and dried flatbreads.

Richard hangs with his wife's friends at parties because he relates better to women. Occasionally, he'll join the husbands and watch the game, commenting on goals scored in basketball and tackles in hockey. He'll say things like, "Aw, *so* close!" and "This is our year!" in a way that's more question than statement. Then, driving home, he'll tell his wife, "I *love* those guys," like he's a real part of the team.

Richard's always smiling in a panicky way that screams,

"Like me! *Please!*" He's dying for acceptance, bends to the tastes of others and constantly seeks approval. It's not that he doesn't know how to be confident, it's that he doesn't know how you *want* him to be confident. Richard's the kind of guy you want to punch in the face and yell, "Be normal, dammit!" but he'd probably praise your right hook. He didn't lose his hair, it abandoned him. Just like his friends and wife will.

If you're reading this book because hair loss has your confidence at an all-time low, you might be a Richard. You're way off the Bald Persona Spectrum because you can't decide who you and your bald head are going to be. As a result, you try to be who you think people want you to be. You're not successful, tough, or mysterious . . . you're Richard, the Bald Pussy whose eyebrows point up in the middle.

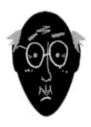

TOM: THE BALD NERD

The saying is, women have to be good-looking while men have to be confident. Makes sense until you look an authentic and unabashed nerd like Tom. Here's someone who's courageous enough to rock the Larry David and blue spectacles, yet Claire, the *Guess Who?* smokeshow, won't even look at him. Something's missing here.

Tom's a nerd's nerd. His raised eyebrows and glazed expression scream, "You're still running a beta point bridge? How's thaaat working for you?" (whatever the fuck that means). He sees the world through a different lens, a higher prescription that makes *Magic: The Gathering* look like *PokerStars*, focusing more on comic conventions than style conventions.

Tom probably puts more stock into his avatar's appearance than his own. He doesn't live in our world and he's happier for it . . . until he sees a girl on a bus who looks like Princess Leah. That's when the hat comes out and insecurity starts to bubble.

If you're a Tom, it's because you choose to be, letting nerd tendencies mold your appearance. In reality, there's no reason why someone who larps has to *look* like someone who larps. There's no reason you can't look good playing *Dungeons and Dragons*.

In 2017, the Toms of the world have hope. Those nerd hobbies aren't so taboo anymore, and with Cosplay and Anime pushing into the mainstream, you can carve out quite the nerd niche. Think of your jump to the Bald Persona Spectrum like a costume you're preparing for a life-long Fan Expo: with some cool glasses, a good haircut and tan—not to mention your sexy gamer skills—you could crush it with all those Batgirls and Harley Quinns.

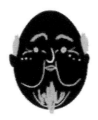

BILL: THE BALD CLOWN

I knew Bill in college. During frosh week, he got so drunk he tried to kick himself in the face.

He broke his leg.

Bill tries to make up for his physical shortcomings by hiding behind a big personality and even bigger antics. He's got the size and stature of The Kingpin but chooses to be Chris Farley; the first of his many lifetime mistakes.

Look at that red face. He's a hall of fame alcoholic.

Like Richard, Bill's persona is the product of low self-esteem and the desire to be liked. However, he's not some impotent worm. Rather, he's a loud, sloppy-joe train wreck that doesn't quit, struggling to one-up his every performance.

Bill will be quick to tell you about the girl who gave him a "blumpkin". Then, while he's telling you what a blumpkin is, you'll realize he told you the same blumpkin story last week. Richard sees him as some kind of football-jersey-wearing deity passing down Greek legends. Others see him as an obvious virgin who cries when he's alone.

Now, being the Big Bald Guy isn't necessarily about being fat. It's about being *that* guy, the one with the big personality and swollen liver.

Only a few people get to see Bill's vulnerable side. He'll drink too much and hunker down on the bathroom floor, talking about his insecurities like he's actually tried facing them. He'll complain to Richard—the only person who can't see through him—that people don't know the "real" him without acknowledging he's never been himself.

Bill is someone who understands the principles of the Bald Persona Spectrum—amplifying certain traits to fit an attractive archetype—but he's way off-base, thinking Homer Simpson is one of the corners.

Never disrespect the BPS.

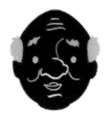

HERMAN: THE BALD WEIRD GUY

Herman doesn't say much, just floats in the background making disingenuous expressions, looking like an empty vessel. You see him at parties but never really meet. He doesn't get texts or emails, but always manages to show up, loitering around. Who invited him? Are you sure he's with us? Is his name even Herman?

His presence alone bums you out. You wonder if even he realizes his irrelevance. What does the world look like through the eyes of an extra?

There's something about him that screams, "always an uncle, never a dad," except he's an uncle you'd never trust with your children.

Making the Leap

You might think the Bald Persona Spectrum is a flawed system because it relies heavily on individual rationalization. I admit it's not perfect. I mean, how well-off can a guy be when he's basing his every move on Dhalsim from *Street Fighter*?

You're right and wrong. Right in that the BPS relies on rationalization but wrong that it's flawed.

The BPS relies on your own personal honesty. If you can look yourself in the mirror and say without a sliver of doubt that you've overcome your hair loss, you'll find a place for yourself within those four corners. There's no quantitative data, no metrics that determine someone's place on the Spectrum. It simply comes down to one question: is balding holding you back?

When I attended the University of Toronto, I took a course called *Urban Sites and Sounds* with a teacher we'll call Prof. The course taught me about semiotics, perspective, and urban space, but most importantly, it proved that a skinny bald man with glasses can own a room.

Prof had a hamster's face with beady eyes and thick hipster glasses, a vague moustache and the stubbled shadow of a receding hairline. Ultimately though, he was bald by choice. He also had these nerd mannerisms and the kind of ambiguous tone that made you wonder: *Did I just make a good point or is he fucking with me in front of the whole class?*

Prof didn't have any of the physical tools to be intimidating or the looks to be captivating, yet he still managed to hook everyone into believing some of the most Freudian bullshit this side of *Inception*. All the girls wanted him and all the guys wanted to be like him. He carried himself with a swagger that would make rappers self-conscious, and it worked because it was unmistakably authentic.

It's easy to picture how Prof could have been a bald nerd like Tom, but something happened. Maybe on his 18th birthday he got his nose pierced and a forearm tattoo after graduation. Then, maybe he enrolled in some psychedelic arts philosophy program and before you knew it . . . he was Dhalsim.

These days, creeping him on the internet, I realize he's not Dhalsim. I don't know who he is but I do know he's got a spot on the BPS. I could get all abstract with what it means to be successful or bend the meaning of tough. One way or another, he'd be there because he wipes his ass with hair loss. He's left his hair in the dust and has overcome his balding.

He's *flourishing*.

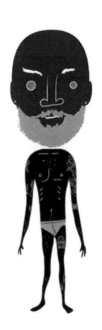

FLOUR-ISH

verb

"to develop in a healthy or successful way"

That Bass

I need to tell you something.

To this point I've been totally honest with you, sometimes to a fault. I've over-shared, told you things, maybe, you didn't need to know.

Sorry, Mom.

I've let you in on some of my darkest thoughts . . . but still, there's a section of my closet that remains cluttered.

It's time to let you know . . . I'm all about that bass.

Maybe it's because I dated a seventy-pound Asian girl through high school? Maybe I saw too much Rachel Ray on TV as a child? Maybe the ass revival and the trailblazers behind it are to blame? Has Nicki Minaj made me this way?

Over time, I've had the courage to come out to a few close friends who were more than supportive. Surprisingly, I wasn't met with ridicule or looks of disgust. In fact, many of them opened up, sharing my affliction, my affinity.

We've all been raised on a standard of beauty is defined by the media. So why—when models and magazine covers sport sleek edges and flat stomachs—is Kat Dennings the first pick in my fantasy draft? How is it that while #thighgap was trending, BBW (Big Beautiful Women) porn was being watched by more people than ever? According to stats published by *PornHub.com*, BBW porn views skyrocketed between 2013 and 2015 by 47%.

Why is it then that a good-looking man with a bigger girl gets rubber-necked like some car accident?

I'm not saying stats from a porn site offer an honest look

into human behavior, but don't they reveal what we're attracted to privately versus publicly?

I don't believe the media dictates beauty standards, I think its radio top forty in a world full of indie heads, punk rockers, thugs, and rednecks, playing what's tried and true while we listen to our own playlists on headphones.

There's no porn category for bald men and there's no one singing, "I'm All About That Bald", but it doesn't mean we're without our own underground community of bald admirers.

So, next time you're getting ready for the club, think twice about grabbing your hat. Maybe the girl you're drooling over's a closeted bald-chaser, tired of hearing '*Tall, Dark and Handsome*' on repeat, and you're hiding your greatest asset.

Men have never understood women, so why start now, believing you know what they find attractive? Instead of reading all the bullshit *Cosmo* surveys and quizzes, take a look around. There are bald men snagging amazing women. Put your head on display and help them find you.

******

The Bald Persona Spectrum and the *Guess Who?* Paradigm are in no way fixed or limiting, and you may find yourself floating between points as you decide who to be. George St Pierre, the UFC legend, is an example of someone who encompasses the breadth of the BPS, with Lex Luthor's wealth, Stone Cold's fight, MJ's athleticism and Dhalsim's aura. Comedian, Joe Rogan would be the same.

When I first began losing my hair, I saw myself as a

reluctant Tom, tall and lanky with pale skin and glasses. I was also friends with a couple of Toms who always bailed on campus parties to "start their own party," which almost always involved video games, frozen pizza, and a black light.

You are who you surround yourself with.

This wasn't the vision of college I saw in the movies, and with my rapidly diminishing hair, I watched that vision slip further and further away. Pandering to the cool kids, I became a skinny Bill, drowning my insecurities with alcohol and masking my discomfort with a big, belligerent personality.

Being Bill generated some good stories, but the acceptance (or self-acceptance) I was looking for was nowhere to be found.

I didn't jump from the *Guess Who?* Paradigm to the Bald Personal Spectrum on purpose. In fact, I came up with them after the fact.

As a second-year art student I became aware of the low-ceiling career options that would be awaiting me after graduation. Coupled with a sense of rebellion against my peers and profs, I started looking for a way out. This lead to the world of tattoos and an apprenticeship at a shop in my home town.

Overnight, people started treating me differently; listening to my stories and asking about designs, hanging on every word with wide-eyed astonishment. I'd spent most of my life as a closeted artist, eventually dabbling in music 'cause drawing was nerd-shit and guitar was punk rock. Still, it wasn't until I wore my art on my sleeve—literally and figuratively—that people started taking notice.

By the time buzzing my head became part of my weekly routine, I was tattooing full-time, with black plugs in my ears and a half-dozen tats of my own. The more hair I lost the more grew on my face, like a beard was my body's defense mechanism to keep me from looking like a tape worm.

Tattooing pulled me from my tailspin and more than made up for the confidence I'd lost balding. Spectrum-wise, I saw myself floating south-southeast, but more importantly I saw myself as more than just a bald head.

I remember a guy from high school coming into the shop, looking for some meat-head design. His name was Brad, the kind of "cool guy" who rolled his shoulders when he walked and tore off his shirt to fight. He opened with, "Brooo, I'm lookin' to get inked," not 'cause he recognized me, but because everyone was bro. Everyone who mattered was bro.

"Check it," he said. "I wanna get my last name written in, like . . . fuckin' stone, with like, broken chains an' shit. You know, like my name's breakin' outta the chains, right? I want it, like, shoulder to shoulder, so, like, it's gonna be pretty big cuz' I've got *broad* shoulders."

Even if I looked the same, douche-Brad wouldn't have recognized me. The old me, balding me, would have gone full Richard, pandering like a schoolgirl. "That sounds sick!" I'd say, scattering a few "fucks" and "shits", like, "That's gonna be some fuckin' cool shit, bro," desperate for some sort of bond with this superior being, this lunkheaded, self-sucking, loser.

But this wasn't the old me. This wasn't Richard, Bill, or Herman. This was The Rock. This was Heisenberg. I crossed my arms and said, "Cool. Is your last name *Douchebag*?"

Years ago, I *looked* like a Tom but didn't *feel* like it. Conjuring Bill's over-the-top personality took more than it was worth, and for a while, I thought I'd end up like Herman.

You can throw a dart at the BPS and choose some bold personality, but that's how you wind up "peacocking"—wearing a costume, reciting lines to get your foot in the door, only to realize you have no idea what to do once you're in. The BPS is about identifying strengths and using them as the foundation of your character, a foundation so strong that hair-loss will never knock you down.

I built my foundation on my artistic talent and pushed that confidence to the front of my character. I moved on from tattooing in 2014 but I still approach every situation as though it were a tattoo consultation. Every conversation takes place in my imaginary studio, in my wheelhouse, where I am skilled and I am validated.

What do all corners of the BPS have in common? Confidence. Passion. Determination. Talent. Traits that inspire, make impact, and leave a lasting impression.

With A Little Help From My Friends

Ding Dong

Adam steps back and adjusts his hat. John fidgets with a string of lights wrapped around his waist while I struggle to see through my mask.

It's Halloween, 2003, and my friends and I are dressed as an entertainment system. Dave's a remote, John's an Xbox, Adam's a DVD player, and I'm a TV.

The wait at the doorstep is long. They've been getting longer as the night's gone on and the number of trick-or-treaters dwindles. People are turning out their lights and my friends and I are some of the last kids going strong. My pillowcase is heavy and my forearms burn. The cardboard box on my head is damp and droopy from the rain, but I persevere.

Most kids bail on halloween at eleven years old, but not me. As an elder trick-or-treater at the ripe age of thirteen, I have the body to hit twice as many houses, carry twice the load, and get twice as much candy. I'm in my halloween prime, I'd be foolish to hang it up!

A light comes on and we stand at attention.

"Trick or . . ."

The door opens and we trail off into slouched mumbles. Standing in the doorway is Jen, easily one of the hottest girls in our grade. Needless to say she wasn't dressed like a PlayStation.

Jen sort of smirks and makes that sour face you make when someone wipes out.

"Free candy! Weeeooo!" shouts John, trying to play the fun guy.

"John!" Dave grunts. "Shut up!"

I couldn't take my eyes from the ground as Jen made her donations. The bite-sized Twix cut through my heart and almost echoed as it hit the bottom of my pillowcase.

What the fuck am I doing? I'm a teenager! I just spent three hours fighting through the rain for a few bite-sized Twix? I have a part time job! I can buy full-sized Twix and not even feel it!

It took me twenty seconds to turn on Halloween, a day I looked forward to for almost an entire decade. How could I be sure of anything anymore?

These days, comparatively, I embrace being bald. But just like my favorite day of the year, my positivity can wane.

Take this week for example. Trent, my co-worker, finally gave into the accounting girls and wore his hair naturally, skipping the flat-iron and rocking his curls. It was a total hit and people are pretty excited about it. I'm happy for Trent, but it's tough to see what a hairstyle can do when the option isn't available to me.

Sure, I can grow a bread and I can put on glasses, but I can't slick back my hair or let it hang in my face. I don't have the option of reinventing myself with a few snips of the scissors. This is what I look like today, and I'll look like this tomorrow.

I'm never gonna be the guy whose wavy locks make girls swoon, and I'm never gonna be the silver fox who can still wheel freshmen. I'm watching *The Bachelorette* and there is zero representation from the bald community — *that says something*. Even when I overcome these things 90% of the time, there's still that 10% that comes as a total gut-punch.

For the most part, I used to push that shit down. I'd look around and think, "Well at least I don't have that guy's acne." I'd pump myself up and think, "I'm the tallest guy on the streetcar, at least I've got that going for me." Sometimes I'd assume attractive people must have shitty character and God doesn't give with both hands. I could tell myself over and over again that all good-looking people have no depth, but it's a momentary solution, a quick high with a long comedown.

Nowadays, I think of the man on the bike.

I was walking to work one day and felt like everyone was looking at me. I imagined each person wondering if I was a young looking old guy, or an old looking young guy. Neither were ideal. I wondered if the sidewalk were a bar, which woman, if any, would be open for a drink? Just as I considered how low that number may be, I heard a bell.

Ring ring!

I looked to my left as a guy whizzed past on a red bicycle. He wore a white tank, exposing his thin arms and various tattoos. Like me, he had a red beard that climbed the sides of his face, giving way to a shaved head. He looked at me through his sunglasses, and almost in slow motion gave me a down-nod.

While an up-nod says, "What's up?" or "Hey!", a down-nod says, "I know" or "I understand". In this instance, the down-nod was a confirmation of solidarity. It said, "I know where your head's at, I've been there too. We all face it, and we all prevail. I got you."

I nodded back.

The man on the bike represents the support you'll have from me and every other bald man you meet. We've all faced it and we've all prevailed. If I'm at a party and I don't know anyone, point me to a bald guy and I'll have a friend. That solidarity, that team approach, is what gets me through the bad days.

******

When I was fourteen, know what I did on October 31st? I dressed up like Santa Claus. John was Batman, Adam was a ghost, and Dave was a pirate. We threw our pillowcases over our shoulders, and we fucking trick-or-treated.

The Butterfly Effect

Halloween looks a little different at 27.

I've moved on from costume club nights to low-key hangouts that wrap up by midnight. I'll admit, the skimpy costumes are a draw, but these days I won't give up sleep for anything less than nipple.

That said, I never pass up the chance to flex my creativity with an outside-the-box costume.

This year, I went as a testimonial for hair plugs. I printed a branded shirt and bought a ridiculous auburn wig. Put the two together and you get "A Man with a New Lease on Life".

As I styled my wig, I fell into a left side sweep. A few more swoops and I rediscovered the *Weber*, the last style I wore by choice, not necessity.

While my face now hides beneath a bushy beard, there was no mistaking my former self looking back in the mirror. I was surprised to see him, but more surprised by how he looked.

Terrible.

The wig irritated my forehead and got in my eyes, forcing me into that old habit of cranking my neck to whip my bangs to the side. My beard and hair clashed, framing my face like a pale-faced lion with a ginger mane.

I realized there's no way I would have grown a beard had I held onto my hair.

You've heard of the Butterfly Effect, where a butterfly flaps it's wings in Mexico and it causes a hurricane in China? It means huge events can be the result of small changes—like a single shed hair.

So what happens to my sense of masculinity if I never grow a beard? What else do I indirectly owe to my bald head?

Obviously, I needed to go bald to write this book. The book helped set me apart while interviewing for my current job. My job allowed me to move closer to my family. Now, I'm able to see my newborn nephew once a week. Can I thank my bald head for that?

It's easy to dream about that hair life, with your products and gels. You'd wear suits and be totally *GQ*, right? You'd drink *Perrier* and have affairs with temps. Maybe that's true, but maybe, like me, you focused on personal development when balding set in. Maybe that influenced you to get serious about guitar. Maybe that kept the band together and lead you to play that show where you met that girl.

******

There's a load of negatives when it comes to being bald, but they often present positive counterpoints. For example, I can't be in on the trendiest hairstyles. Counterpoint? I save a shitload of money on cuts and products. I'll never embarrass myself with a man-bun or top-knot. I never have to worry about my look holding up in the rain, and humidity is a total non-factor.

Recently, I was at a bar with my friend and our waitress guessed I was thirty-five, despite actually being twenty-seven. I didn't go running to the mall in a panic, stocking up on graphic tees and hoodies, I stayed composed and tried to find the counterpoints.

1) Looking older isn't always bad. The waitress said I looked thirty-five, not sixty-five, and plenty of women think thirty's a man's prime. Notice I said 'man' and not 'boy'. Really, who cares about some nineteen-year-old who'd bitch about my Facebook status? Haven't I moved passed girls and on to women?

2) Even if I do look a decade older, I could look this good for the next thirty years. With hair loss already behind me, *I'll* be the lady killer, head held high, when my slouched peers start counting hairs on their pillows.

That's another thing, most guys will go bald in their forties and fifties. In fact, by thirty-five, two out of three men are thinning, and by fifty, most have experienced significant hair loss.

Once you go through it, it's almost like gaining a super power—the ability to see the bald future before anyone else. Every day, I notice hairlines and crop circles on the subway and sidewalk. I used to know a girl named Brittany, who tried getting under my skin by taking shots at my bald head. I wouldn't fire back. Instead, I laughed and brushed it off, knowing her boyfriend was two years away from being a fellow baldy. She just didn't know it yet.

I wonder if they're still together?

Speaking of couples, my girlfriend, Kelly, serves as a daily reminder that balding hasn't held me back one bit. Although I started the relationship with an inconspicuous sweep, she's literally stuck by me through thick and thin. While my former boss's wife forbids him from shaving his head, Kelly's been supportive and actually encouraged me to tap out.

"It suits you," she says. "You look tougher, more confident."

In the same way I see my Dad, Kelly can't picture me with hair anymore, and thankfully, that version's been long forgotten. One of my friends recalls wanting to punch the me in the face when we first met, saying my hair made me *super punchable*. I can't disagree, looking back at old photos I'd punch that swoop-banged shit-head too.

So, how do I see myself now?

These days, I try to avoid saying I'm bald, instead choosing to say I shave my head. To me, "bald" has a negative connotation that doesn't apply anymore. I may not have hair, but that doesn't make me bald.

Years ago, I remember getting off the bus on my way to work. This guy, Nathan, was waiting for me at my bus stop. I'd been tattooing his girlfriend fairly regularly and he was convinced we were hooking up behind his back. He'd taken a two-hour bus ride to shake me down.

"Dude," I laughed. "I'm twenty-four and going bald. Are you seriously threatened by me?

He held his ground, snarling like he was really gonna do something. I brushed by and signaled for him to follow. For the next block, I gave Nathan some relationship advice. He wasn't smart, wasn't funny, and didn't have a promising future. The only thing he had was a girlfriend who could do better . . . and he knew it.

Despite having a full head of thick, wavy hair, deep down, Nathan was bald. The panic I saw in his eyes reminded me of the *old* me, counting hairs on my pillow, angry and afraid, fighting to regain the control I never had to begin with.

That's when I was bald.

I was bald when I saw Joan as wifey material. I was bald when I was shopping for extra virgin olive oil. I was bald in my shitty dorm washroom, marking my forehead in sharpie.

I'm not that guy anymore.

Who's bald? The overly-possessive boyfriend is bald. The guy who wears his t-shirt in the pool is bald. The guy who deserves a raise but doesn't have the balls to ask for it is bald. The comb-over's bald. Hats are bald. The hair growth pills, the medication, the plugs . . . they're all fucking bald!

The truth about hair loss is that it starts on your head and finishes in your head. It's not a bad haircut, it's a bad state of mind, a negative view of your self-worth. And as soon as you realize that, you'll realize it can't hold you back.

In the words of George Costanza, a man who—despite getting fucked on height, weight, vision, and hair—got a job with the Yankees and had sex with the cleaning woman on his desk.

"I'm not bald. I *was* bald."

What did you think of this story?

Head over to www.bookofbald.com and give a review.